BLOOD PRESSURE LOG

NAME. ___________________________

Date	AM		PM		Notes
	Blood pressure	Pulse	Blood pressure	Pulse	

Level of Severity	Systolic	Diastolic
Normal	120	80
Mild Hypertension	140-160	90-100
Moderate Hypertension	160-200	100-120
Severe Hypertension	Above 200	160-200

Blood Pressure Log

NAME. ____

Date	AM		PM		Notes
	Blood pressure	Pulse	Blood pressure	Pulse	

Level of Severity	Systolic	Diastolic
Normal	120	80
Mild Hypertension	140-160	90-100
Moderate Hypertension	160-200	100-120
Severe Hypertension	Above 200	160-200

BLOOD PRESSURE LOG

NAME. ____

Date	AM		PM		Notes
	Blood pressure	Pulse	Blood pressure	Pulse	

Level of Severity	Systolic	Diastolic
Normal	120	80
Mild Hypertension	140-160	90-100
Moderate Hypertension	160-200	100-120
Severe Hypertension	Above 200	160-200

BLOOD PRESSURE LOG

NAME. ____

Date	AM		PM		Notes
	Blood pressure	Pulse	Blood pressure	Pulse	

Level of Severity	Systolic	Diastolic
Normal	120	80
Mild Hypertension	140-160	90-100
Moderate Hypertension	160-200	100-120
Severe Hypertension	Above 200	160-200

BLOOD PRESSURE LOG

NAME. ___________________________________

Date	AM		PM		Notes
	Blood pressure	Pulse	Blood pressure	Pulse	

Level of Severity	Systolic	Diastolic
Normal	120	80
Mild Hypertension	140-160	90-100
Moderate Hypertension	160-200	100-120
Severe Hypertension	Above 200	160-200

BLOOD PRESSURE LOG

NAME. ____

Date	AM		PM		Notes
	Blood pressure	Pulse	Blood pressure	Pulse	

Level of Severity	Systolic	Diastolic
Normal	120	80
Mild Hypertension	140-160	90-100
Moderate Hypertension	160-200	100-120
Severe Hypertension	Above 200	160-200

BLOOD PRESSURE LOG

NAME. ____

Date	AM		PM		Notes
	Blood pressure	Pulse	Blood pressure	Pulse	

vel of Severity	Systolic	Diastolic
rmal	120	80
d Hypertension	140-160	90-100
derate Hypertension	160-200	100-120
vere Hypertension	Above 200	160-200

BLOOD PRESSURE LOG

NAME. ____

Date	AM		PM		Notes
	Blood pressure	Pulse	Blood pressure	Pulse	

Level of Severity	Systolic	Diastolic
Normal	120	80
Mild Hypertension	140-160	90-100
Moderate Hypertension	160-200	100-120
Severe Hypertension	Above 200	160-200

BLOOD PRESSURE LOG

NAME. ____

Date	AM		PM		Notes
	Blood pressure	Pulse	Blood pressure	Pulse	

Level of Severity	Systolic	Diastolic
Normal	120	80
Mild Hypertension	140-160	90-100
Moderate Hypertension	160-200	100-120
Severe Hypertension	Above 200	160-200

Blood Pressure Log

NAME. ____

Date	AM		PM		Notes
	Blood pressure	Pulse	Blood pressure	Pulse	

Level of Severity	Systolic	Diastolic
Normal	120	80
Mild Hypertension	140-160	90-100
Moderate Hypertension	160-200	100-120
Severe Hypertension	Above 200	160-200

BLOOD PRESSURE LOG

NAME. _______________________________

Date	AM		PM		Notes
	Blood pressure	Pulse	Blood pressure	Pulse	

Level of Severity	Systolic	Diastolic
Normal	120	80
Mild Hypertension	140-160	90-100
Moderate Hypertension	160-200	100-120
Severe Hypertension	Above 200	160-200

BLOOD PRESSURE LOG

NAME. ____

Date	AM		PM		Notes
	Blood pressure	Pulse	Blood pressure	Pulse	

Level of Severity	Systolic	Diastolic
Normal	120	80
Mild Hypertension	140-160	90-100
Moderate Hypertension	160-200	100-120
Severe Hypertension	Above 200	160-200

BLOOD PRESSURE LOG

NAME. _______________________________

Date	AM		PM		Notes
	Blood pressure	Pulse	Blood pressure	Pulse	

vel of Severity	Systolic	Diastolic
rmal	120	80
d Hypertension	140-160	90-100
derate Hypertension	160-200	100-120
vere Hypertension	Above 200	160-200

BLOOD PRESSURE LOG

NAME. ____

Date	AM		PM		Notes
	Blood pressure	Pulse	Blood pressure	Pulse	

Level of Severity	Systolic	Diastolic
Normal	120	80
Mild Hypertension	140-160	90-100
Moderate Hypertension	160-200	100-120
Severe Hypertension	Above 200	160-200

BLOOD PRESSURE LOG

NAME. ____

Date	AM		PM		Notes
	Blood pressure	Pulse	Blood pressure	Pulse	

Level of Severity	Systolic	Diastolic
Normal	120	80
Mild Hypertension	140-160	90-100
Moderate Hypertension	160-200	100-120
Severe Hypertension	Above 200	160-200

BLOOD PRESSURE LOG

NAME. ____

Date	AM		PM		Notes
	Blood pressure	Pulse	Blood pressure	Pulse	

Level of Severity	Systolic	Diastolic
Normal	120	80
Mild Hypertension	140-160	90-100
Moderate Hypertension	160-200	100-120
Severe Hypertension	Above 200	160-200

Blood Pressure Log

NAME. ______________________________

Date	AM		PM		Notes
	Blood pressure	Pulse	Blood pressure	Pulse	

Level of Severity	Systolic	Diastolic
Normal	120	80
Mild Hypertension	140-160	90-100
Moderate Hypertension	160-200	100-120
Severe Hypertension	Above 200	160-200

BLOOD PRESSURE LOG

NAME. ____

Date	AM		PM		Notes
	Blood pressure	Pulse	Blood pressure	Pulse	

Level of Severity	Systolic	Diastolic
Normal	120	80
Mild Hypertension	140-160	90-100
Moderate Hypertension	160-200	100-120
Severe Hypertension	Above 200	160-200

BLOOD PRESSURE LOG

NAME. ____

Date	AM		PM		Notes
	Blood pressure	Pulse	Blood pressure	Pulse	

vel of Severity	Systolic	Diastolic
rmal	120	80
d Hypertension	140-160	90-100
derate Hypertension	160-200	100-120
vere Hypertension	Above 200	160-200

BLOOD PRESSURE LOG

NAME. ____

Date	AM		PM		Notes
	Blood pressure	Pulse	Blood pressure	Pulse	

Level of Severity	Systolic	Diastolic
Normal	120	80
Mild Hypertension	140-160	90-100
Moderate Hypertension	160-200	100-120
Severe Hypertension	Above 200	160-200

BLOOD PRESSURE LOG

NAME. _______________________________

Date	AM		PM		Notes
	Blood pressure	Pulse	Blood pressure	Pulse	

Level of Severity	Systolic	Diastolic
Normal	120	80
Mild Hypertension	140-160	90-100
Moderate Hypertension	160-200	100-120
Severe Hypertension	Above 200	160-200

Blood Pressure Log

Name. ___________________________________

Date	AM		PM		Notes
	Blood pressure	Pulse	Blood pressure	Pulse	

Level of Severity	Systolic	Diastolic
Normal	120	80
Mild Hypertension	140-160	90-100
Moderate Hypertension	160-200	100-120
Severe Hypertension	Above 200	160-200

BLOOD PRESSURE LOG

NAME. ____

Date	AM		PM		Notes
	Blood pressure	Pulse	Blood pressure	Pulse	

Level of Severity	Systolic	Diastolic
Normal	120	80
Mild Hypertension	140-160	90-100
Moderate Hypertension	160-200	100-120
Severe Hypertension	Above 200	160-200

BLOOD PRESSURE LOG

NAME. ____

Date	AM		PM		Notes
	Blood pressure	Pulse	Blood pressure	Pulse	

Level of Severity	Systolic	Diastolic
Normal	120	80
Mild Hypertension	140-160	90-100
Moderate Hypertension	160-200	100-120
Severe Hypertension	Above 200	160-200

BLOOD PRESSURE LOG

NAME. ____

Date	AM		PM		Notes
	Blood pressure	Pulse	Blood pressure	Pulse	

vel of Severity	Systolic	Diastolic
rmal	120	80
d Hypertension	140-160	90-100
derate Hypertension	160-200	100-120
vere Hypertension	Above 200	160-200

BLOOD PRESSURE LOG

NAME. ____

Date	AM		PM		Notes
	Blood pressure	Pulse	Blood pressure	Pulse	

Level of Severity	Systolic	Diastolic
Normal	120	80
Mild Hypertension	140-160	90-100
Moderate Hypertension	160-200	100-120
Severe Hypertension	Above 200	160-200

BLOOD PRESSURE LOG

NAME. ____

Date	AM		PM		Notes
	Blood pressure	Pulse	Blood pressure	Pulse	

Level of Severity	Systolic	Diastolic
Normal	120	80
Mild Hypertension	140-160	90-100
Moderate Hypertension	160-200	100-120
Severe Hypertension	Above 200	160-200

Blood Pressure Log

NAME. ____

Date	AM		PM		Notes
	Blood pressure	Pulse	Blood pressure	Pulse	

Level of Severity	Systolic	Diastolic
Normal	120	80
Mild Hypertension	140-160	90-100
Moderate Hypertension	160-200	100-120
Severe Hypertension	Above 200	160-200

BLOOD PRESSURE LOG

NAME. ____

Date	AM		PM		Notes
	Blood pressure	Pulse	Blood pressure	Pulse	

Level of Severity	Systolic	Diastolic
Normal	120	80
Mild Hypertension	140-160	90-100
Moderate Hypertension	160-200	100-120
Severe Hypertension	Above 200	160-200

Blood Pressure Log

NAME. ____

Date	AM		PM		Notes
	Blood pressure	Pulse	Blood pressure	Pulse	

Level of Severity	Systolic	Diastolic
Normal	120	80
Mild Hypertension	140-160	90-100
Moderate Hypertension	160-200	100-120
Severe Hypertension	Above 200	160-200

BLOOD PRESSURE LOG

NAME. ______________________________

Date	AM		PM		Notes
	Blood pressure	Pulse	Blood pressure	Pulse	

Level of Severity	Systolic	Diastolic
Normal	120	80
Mild Hypertension	140-160	90-100
Moderate Hypertension	160-200	100-120
Severe Hypertension	Above 200	160-200

BLOOD PRESSURE LOG

NAME. ____

Date	AM		PM		Notes
	Blood pressure	Pulse	Blood pressure	Pulse	

Level of Severity	Systolic	Diastolic
Normal	120	80
Mild Hypertension	140-160	90-100
Moderate Hypertension	160-200	100-120
Severe Hypertension	Above 200	160-200

BLOOD PRESSURE LOG

NAME. _______________________________

Date	AM		PM		Notes
	Blood pressure	Pulse	Blood pressure	Pulse	

Level of Severity	Systolic	Diastolic
Normal	120	80
Mild Hypertension	140-160	90-100
Moderate Hypertension	160-200	100-120
Severe Hypertension	Above 200	160-200

BLOOD PRESSURE LOG

NAME. ____

Date	AM		PM		Notes
	Blood pressure	Pulse	Blood pressure	Pulse	

Level of Severity	Systolic	Diastolic
Normal	120	80
Mild Hypertension	140-160	90-100
Moderate Hypertension	160-200	100-120
Severe Hypertension	Above 200	160-200

BLOOD PRESSURE LOG

NAME. ___________________________________

Date	AM		PM		Notes
	Blood pressure	Pulse	Blood pressure	Pulse	

Level of Severity	Systolic	Diastolic
Normal	120	80
Mild Hypertension	140-160	90-100
Moderate Hypertension	160-200	100-120
Severe Hypertension	Above 200	160-200

BLOOD PRESSURE LOG

NAME. ____

Date	AM		PM		Notes
	Blood pressure	Pulse	Blood pressure	Pulse	

Level of Severity	Systolic	Diastolic
Normal	120	80
Mild Hypertension	140-160	90-100
Moderate Hypertension	160-200	100-120
Severe Hypertension	Above 200	160-200

BLOOD PRESSURE LOG

NAME. ______________________________

Date	AM		PM		Notes
	Blood pressure	Pulse	Blood pressure	Pulse	

vel of Severity	Systolic	Diastolic
rmal	120	80
d Hypertension	140-160	90-100
derate Hypertension	160-200	100-120
vere Hypertension	Above 200	160-200

BLOOD PRESSURE LOG

NAME. ____

Date	AM		PM		Notes
	Blood pressure	Pulse	Blood pressure	Pulse	

Level of Severity	Systolic	Diastolic
Normal	120	80
Mild Hypertension	140-160	90-100
Moderate Hypertension	160-200	100-120
Severe Hypertension	Above 200	160-200

BLOOD PRESSURE LOG

NAME. ___________________________________

Date	AM		PM		Notes
	Blood pressure	Pulse	Blood pressure	Pulse	

Level of Severity	Systolic	Diastolic
Normal	120	80
Mild Hypertension	140-160	90-100
Moderate Hypertension	160-200	100-120
Severe Hypertension	Above 200	160-200

Blood Pressure Log

NAME. ____

Date	AM		PM		Notes
	Blood pressure	Pulse	Blood pressure	Pulse	

Level of Severity	Systolic	Diastolic
Normal	120	80
Mild Hypertension	140-160	90-100
Moderate Hypertension	160-200	100-120
Severe Hypertension	Above 200	160-200

BLOOD PRESSURE LOG

NAME. ____

Date	AM		PM		Notes
	Blood pressure	Pulse	Blood pressure	Pulse	

Level of Severity	Systolic	Diastolic
Normal	120	80
Mild Hypertension	140-160	90-100
Moderate Hypertension	160-200	100-120
Severe Hypertension	Above 200	160-200

BLOOD PRESSURE LOG

NAME. ____

Date	AM		PM		Notes
	Blood pressure	Pulse	Blood pressure	Pulse	

Level of Severity	Systolic	Diastolic
Normal	120	80
Mild Hypertension	140-160	90-100
Moderate Hypertension	160-200	100-120
Severe Hypertension	Above 200	160-200

Blood Pressure Log

Name. ____

Date	AM		PM		Notes
	Blood pressure	Pulse	Blood pressure	Pulse	

Level of Severity	Systolic	Diastolic
Normal	120	80
Mild Hypertension	140-160	90-100
Moderate Hypertension	160-200	100-120
Severe Hypertension	Above 200	160-200

BLOOD PRESSURE LOG

NAME. ____

Date	AM		PM		Notes
	Blood pressure	Pulse	Blood pressure	Pulse	

Level of Severity	Systolic	Diastolic
Normal	120	80
Mild Hypertension	140-160	90-100
Moderate Hypertension	160-200	100-120
Severe Hypertension	Above 200	160-200

BLOOD PRESSURE LOG

NAME. ____

Date	AM		PM		Notes
	Blood pressure	Pulse	Blood pressure	Pulse	

vel of Severity	Systolic	Diastolic
ormal	120	80
ld Hypertension	140-160	90-100
oderate Hypertension	160-200	100-120
evere Hypertension	Above 200	160-200

Blood Pressure Log

NAME. ____

Date	AM		PM		Notes
	Blood pressure	Pulse	Blood pressure	Pulse	

Level of Severity	Systolic	Diastolic
Normal	120	80
Mild Hypertension	140-160	90-100
Moderate Hypertension	160-200	100-120
Severe Hypertension	Above 200	160-200

BLOOD PRESSURE LOG

NAME. _______________________________

Date	AM		PM		Notes
	Blood pressure	Pulse	Blood pressure	Pulse	

Level of Severity	Systolic	Diastolic
Normal	120	80
Mild Hypertension	140-160	90-100
Moderate Hypertension	160-200	100-120
Severe Hypertension	Above 200	160-200

BLOOD PRESSURE LOG

NAME. ____

Date	AM		PM		Notes
	Blood pressure	Pulse	Blood pressure	Pulse	

Level of Severity	Systolic	Diastolic
Normal	120	80
Mild Hypertension	140-160	90-100
Moderate Hypertension	160-200	100-120
Severe Hypertension	Above 200	160-200

Blood Pressure Log

NAME. _______________________________

Date	AM		PM		Notes
	Blood pressure	Pulse	Blood pressure	Pulse	

Level of Severity	Systolic	Diastolic
Normal	120	80
Mild Hypertension	140-160	90-100
Moderate Hypertension	160-200	100-120
Severe Hypertension	Above 200	160-200

BLOOD PRESSURE LOG

NAME. ____

Date	AM		PM		Notes
	Blood pressure	Pulse	Blood pressure	Pulse	

Level of Severity	Systolic	Diastolic
Normal	120	80
Mild Hypertension	140-160	90-100
Moderate Hypertension	160-200	100-120
Severe Hypertension	Above 200	160-200

BLOOD PRESSURE LOG

NAME. ____

Date	AM		PM		Notes
	Blood pressure	Pulse	Blood pressure	Pulse	

Level of Severity	Systolic	Diastolic
Normal	120	80
Mild Hypertension	140-160	90-100
Moderate Hypertension	160-200	100-120
Severe Hypertension	Above 200	160-200

BLOOD PRESSURE LOG

NAME. ____

Date	AM		PM		Notes
	Blood pressure	Pulse	Blood pressure	Pulse	

Level of Severity	Systolic	Diastolic
Normal	120	80
Mild Hypertension	140-160	90-100
Moderate Hypertension	160-200	100-120
Severe Hypertension	Above 200	160-200

Blood Pressure Log

Name. ______________________________

Date	AM		PM		Notes
	Blood pressure	Pulse	Blood pressure	Pulse	

Level of Severity	Systolic	Diastolic
Normal	120	80
Mild Hypertension	140-160	90-100
Moderate Hypertension	160-200	100-120
Severe Hypertension	Above 200	160-200

BLOOD PRESSURE LOG

NAME. _______________________________________

Date	AM		PM		Notes
	Blood pressure	Pulse	Blood pressure	Pulse	

Level of Severity	Systolic	Diastolic
Normal	120	80
Mild Hypertension	140-160	90-100
Moderate Hypertension	160-200	100-120
Severe Hypertension	Above 200	160-200

Blood Pressure Log

NAME. ____

Date	AM		PM		Notes
	Blood pressure	Pulse	Blood pressure	Pulse	

vel of Severity	Systolic	Diastolic
rmal	120	80
d Hypertension	140-160	90-100
derate Hypertension	160-200	100-120
vere Hypertension	Above 200	160-200

Blood Pressure Log

NAME. ____

Date	AM		PM		Notes
	Blood pressure	Pulse	Blood pressure	Pulse	

Level of Severity	Systolic	Diastolic
Normal	120	80
Mild Hypertension	140-160	90-100
Moderate Hypertension	160-200	100-120
Severe Hypertension	Above 200	160-200

BLOOD PRESSURE LOG

NAME. ______________________________

Date	AM		PM		Notes
	Blood pressure	Pulse	Blood pressure	Pulse	

vel of Severity	Systolic	Diastolic
rmal	120	80
ld Hypertension	140-160	90-100
oderate Hypertension	160-200	100-120
vere Hypertension	Above 200	160-200

BLOOD PRESSURE LOG

NAME. ____

Date	AM		PM		Notes
	Blood pressure	Pulse	Blood pressure	Pulse	

Level of Severity	Systolic	Diastolic
Normal	120	80
Mild Hypertension	140-160	90-100
Moderate Hypertension	160-200	100-120
Severe Hypertension	Above 200	160-200

BLOOD PRESSURE LOG

NAME. ___________________________

Date	AM		PM		Notes
	Blood pressure	Pulse	Blood pressure	Pulse	

Level of Severity	Systolic	Diastolic
Normal	120	80
Mild Hypertension	140-160	90-100
Moderate Hypertension	160-200	100-120
Severe Hypertension	Above 200	160-200

BLOOD PRESSURE LOG

NAME. ____

Date	AM		PM		Notes
	Blood pressure	Pulse	Blood pressure	Pulse	

Level of Severity	Systolic	Diastolic
Normal	120	80
Mild Hypertension	140-160	90-100
Moderate Hypertension	160-200	100-120
Severe Hypertension	Above 200	160-200

BLOOD PRESSURE LOG

NAME. ____

Date	AM		PM		Notes
	Blood pressure	Pulse	Blood pressure	Pulse	

vel of Severity	Systolic	Diastolic
rmal	120	80
d Hypertension	140-160	90-100
derate Hypertension	160-200	100-120
vere Hypertension	Above 200	160-200

BLOOD PRESSURE LOG

NAME. ____

Date	AM		PM		Notes
	Blood pressure	Pulse	Blood pressure	Pulse	

Level of Severity	Systolic	Diastolic
Normal	120	80
Mild Hypertension	140-160	90-100
Moderate Hypertension	160-200	100-120
Severe Hypertension	Above 200	160-200

BLOOD PRESSURE LOG

NAME. ____

Date	AM		PM		Notes
	Blood pressure	Pulse	Blood pressure	Pulse	

vel of Severity	Systolic	Diastolic
rmal	120	80
ld Hypertension	140-160	90-100
oderate Hypertension	160-200	100-120
vere Hypertension	Above 200	160-200

BLOOD PRESSURE LOG

NAME. ____

Date	AM		PM		Notes
	Blood pressure	Pulse	Blood pressure	Pulse	

Level of Severity	Systolic	Diastolic
Normal	120	80
Mild Hypertension	140-160	90-100
Moderate Hypertension	160-200	100-120
Severe Hypertension	Above 200	160-200

BLOOD PRESSURE LOG

NAME. ____

Date	AM		PM		Notes
	Blood pressure	Pulse	Blood pressure	Pulse	

Level of Severity	Systolic	Diastolic
Normal	120	80
Mild Hypertension	140-160	90-100
Moderate Hypertension	160-200	100-120
Severe Hypertension	Above 200	160-200

BLOOD PRESSURE LOG

NAME. ____

Date	AM		PM		Notes
	Blood pressure	Pulse	Blood pressure	Pulse	

Level of Severity	Systolic	Diastolic
Normal	120	80
Mild Hypertension	140-160	90-100
Moderate Hypertension	160-200	100-120
Severe Hypertension	Above 200	160-200

BLOOD PRESSURE LOG

NAME. ____

Date	AM		PM		Notes
	Blood pressure	Pulse	Blood pressure	Pulse	

el of Severity	Systolic	Diastolic
rmal	120	80
d Hypertension	140-160	90-100
derate Hypertension	160-200	100-120
vere Hypertension	Above 200	160-200

BLOOD PRESSURE LOG

NAME. ____

Date	AM		PM		Notes
	Blood pressure	Pulse	Blood pressure	Pulse	

Level of Severity	Systolic	Diastolic
Normal	120	80
Mild Hypertension	140-160	90-100
Moderate Hypertension	160-200	100-120
Severe Hypertension	Above 200	160-200

BLOOD PRESSURE LOG

NAME. ____

Date	AM		PM		Notes
	Blood pressure	Pulse	Blood pressure	Pulse	

vel of Severity	Systolic	Diastolic
rmal	120	80
ld Hypertension	140-160	90-100
oderate Hypertension	160-200	100-120
vere Hypertension	Above 200	160-200

Blood Pressure Log

NAME. ____

Date	AM		PM		Notes
	Blood pressure	Pulse	Blood pressure	Pulse	

Level of Severity	Systolic	Diastolic
Normal	120	80
Mild Hypertension	140-160	90-100
Moderate Hypertension	160-200	100-120
Severe Hypertension	Above 200	160-200

BLOOD PRESSURE LOG

NAME. ____

Date	AM		PM		Notes
	Blood pressure	Pulse	Blood pressure	Pulse	

Level of Severity	Systolic	Diastolic
Normal	120	80
Mild Hypertension	140-160	90-100
Moderate Hypertension	160-200	100-120
Severe Hypertension	Above 200	160-200

BLOOD PRESSURE LOG

NAME. ____

Date	AM		PM		Notes
	Blood pressure	Pulse	Blood pressure	Pulse	

Level of Severity	Systolic	Diastolic
Normal	120	80
Mild Hypertension	140-160	90-100
Moderate Hypertension	160-200	100-120
Severe Hypertension	Above 200	160-200

Blood Pressure Log

NAME. ______________________________

Date	AM		PM		Notes
	Blood pressure	Pulse	Blood pressure	Pulse	

el of Severity	Systolic	Diastolic
mal	120	80
d Hypertension	140-160	90-100
derate Hypertension	160-200	100-120
vere Hypertension	Above 200	160-200

BLOOD PRESSURE LOG

NAME. ____

Date	AM		PM		Notes
	Blood pressure	Pulse	Blood pressure	Pulse	

Level of Severity	Systolic	Diastolic
Normal	120	80
Mild Hypertension	140-160	90-100
Moderate Hypertension	160-200	100-120
Severe Hypertension	Above 200	160-200

Blood Pressure Log

Name. ________________________________

Date	AM		PM		Notes
	Blood pressure	Pulse	Blood pressure	Pulse	

Level of Severity	Systolic	Diastolic
Normal	120	80
Mild Hypertension	140-160	90-100
Moderate Hypertension	160-200	100-120
Severe Hypertension	Above 200	160-200

BLOOD PRESSURE LOG

NAME. ____

Date	AM		PM		Notes
	Blood pressure	Pulse	Blood pressure	Pulse	

Level of Severity	Systolic	Diastolic
Normal	120	80
Mild Hypertension	140-160	90-100
Moderate Hypertension	160-200	100-120
Severe Hypertension	Above 200	160-200

BLOOD PRESSURE LOG

NAME. ____

Date	AM		PM		Notes
	Blood pressure	Pulse	Blood pressure	Pulse	

Level of Severity	Systolic	Diastolic
Normal	120	80
Mild Hypertension	140-160	90-100
Moderate Hypertension	160-200	100-120
Severe Hypertension	Above 200	160-200

BLOOD PRESSURE LOG

NAME. ____

Date	AM		PM		Notes
	Blood pressure	Pulse	Blood pressure	Pulse	

Level of Severity	Systolic	Diastolic
Normal	120	80
Mild Hypertension	140-160	90-100
Moderate Hypertension	160-200	100-120
Severe Hypertension	Above 200	160-200

BLOOD PRESSURE LOG

NAME. ____

Date	AM		PM		Notes
	Blood pressure	Pulse	Blood pressure	Pulse	

vel of Severity	Systolic	Diastolic
rmal	120	80
d Hypertension	140-160	90-100
derate Hypertension	160-200	100-120
vere Hypertension	Above 200	160-200

Blood Pressure Log

Name. ______________________________________

Date	AM		PM		Notes
	Blood pressure	Pulse	Blood pressure	Pulse	

Level of Severity	Systolic	Diastolic
Normal	120	80
Mild Hypertension	140-160	90-100
Moderate Hypertension	160-200	100-120
Severe Hypertension	Above 200	160-200

BLOOD PRESSURE LOG

NAME. ____

Date	AM		PM		Notes
	Blood pressure	Pulse	Blood pressure	Pulse	

vel of Severity	Systolic	Diastolic
rmal	120	80
ld Hypertension	140-160	90-100
oderate Hypertension	160-200	100-120
vere Hypertension	Above 200	160-200

BLOOD PRESSURE LOG

NAME. ____

Date	AM		PM		Notes
	Blood pressure	Pulse	Blood pressure	Pulse	

Level of Severity	Systolic	Diastolic
Normal	120	80
Mild Hypertension	140-160	90-100
Moderate Hypertension	160-200	100-120
Severe Hypertension	Above 200	160-200

BLOOD PRESSURE LOG

NAME. ____

Date	AM		PM		Notes
	Blood pressure	Pulse	Blood pressure	Pulse	

Level of Severity	Systolic	Diastolic
Normal	120	80
Mild Hypertension	140-160	90-100
Moderate Hypertension	160-200	100-120
Severe Hypertension	Above 200	160-200

BLOOD PRESSURE LOG

NAME. ____

Date	AM		PM		Notes
	Blood pressure	Pulse	Blood pressure	Pulse	

Level of Severity	Systolic	Diastolic
Normal	120	80
Mild Hypertension	140-160	90-100
Moderate Hypertension	160-200	100-120
Severe Hypertension	Above 200	160-200

BLOOD PRESSURE LOG

NAME. ____

Date	AM		PM		Notes
	Blood pressure	Pulse	Blood pressure	Pulse	

vel of Severity	Systolic	Diastolic
rmal	120	80
d Hypertension	140-160	90-100
derate Hypertension	160-200	100-120
vere Hypertension	Above 200	160-200

BLOOD PRESSURE LOG

NAME. ____

Date	AM		PM		Notes
	Blood pressure	Pulse	Blood pressure	Pulse	

Level of Severity	Systolic	Diastolic
Normal	120	80
Mild Hypertension	140-160	90-100
Moderate Hypertension	160-200	100-120
Severe Hypertension	Above 200	160-200

BLOOD PRESSURE LOG

NAME. ____

Date	AM		PM		Notes
	Blood pressure	Pulse	Blood pressure	Pulse	

Level of Severity	Systolic	Diastolic
Normal	120	80
Mild Hypertension	140-160	90-100
Moderate Hypertension	160-200	100-120
Severe Hypertension	Above 200	160-200

Blood Pressure Log

Name. ____

Date	AM		PM		Notes
	Blood pressure	Pulse	Blood pressure	Pulse	

Level of Severity	Systolic	Diastolic
Normal	120	80
Mild Hypertension	140-160	90-100
Moderate Hypertension	160-200	100-120
Severe Hypertension	Above 200	160-200

BLOOD PRESSURE LOG

NAME. ____

Date	AM		PM		Notes
	Blood pressure	Pulse	Blood pressure	Pulse	

Level of Severity	Systolic	Diastolic
Normal	120	80
Mild Hypertension	140-160	90-100
Moderate Hypertension	160-200	100-120
Severe Hypertension	Above 200	160-200

BLOOD PRESSURE LOG

NAME. ____

Date	AM		PM		Notes
	Blood pressure	Pulse	Blood pressure	Pulse	

Level of Severity	Systolic	Diastolic
Normal	120	80
Mild Hypertension	140-160	90-100
Moderate Hypertension	160-200	100-120
Severe Hypertension	Above 200	160-200

Blood Pressure Log

NAME. _______________________________

Date	AM		PM		Notes
	Blood pressure	Pulse	Blood pressure	Pulse	

el of Severity	Systolic	Diastolic
mal	120	80
d Hypertension	140-160	90-100
derate Hypertension	160-200	100-120
ere Hypertension	Above 200	160-200

BLOOD PRESSURE LOG

NAME. ____

Date	AM		PM		Notes
	Blood pressure	Pulse	Blood pressure	Pulse	

Level of Severity	Systolic	Diastolic
Normal	120	80
Mild Hypertension	140-160	90-100
Moderate Hypertension	160-200	100-120
Severe Hypertension	Above 200	160-200

BLOOD PRESSURE LOG

NAME. ____

Date	AM		PM		Notes
	Blood pressure	Pulse	Blood pressure	Pulse	

Level of Severity	Systolic	Diastolic
Normal	120	80
Mild Hypertension	140-160	90-100
Moderate Hypertension	160-200	100-120
Severe Hypertension	Above 200	160-200

Blood Pressure Log

NAME. ____

Date	AM		PM		Notes
	Blood pressure	Pulse	Blood pressure	Pulse	

Level of Severity	Systolic	Diastolic
Normal	120	80
Mild Hypertension	140-160	90-100
Moderate Hypertension	160-200	100-120
Severe Hypertension	Above 200	160-200

BLOOD PRESSURE LOG

NAME. ____

Date	AM		PM		Notes
	Blood pressure	Pulse	Blood pressure	Pulse	

Level of Severity	Systolic	Diastolic
Normal	120	80
Mild Hypertension	140-160	90-100
Moderate Hypertension	160-200	100-120
Severe Hypertension	Above 200	160-200

BLOOD PRESSURE LOG

NAME. ____

Date	AM		PM		Notes
	Blood pressure	Pulse	Blood pressure	Pulse	

Level of Severity	Systolic	Diastolic
Normal	120	80
Mild Hypertension	140-160	90-100
Moderate Hypertension	160-200	100-120
Severe Hypertension	Above 200	160-200

BLOOD PRESSURE LOG

NAME. ____

Date	AM		PM		Notes
	Blood pressure	Pulse	Blood pressure	Pulse	

el of Severity	Systolic	Diastolic
mal	120	80
d Hypertension	140-160	90-100
derate Hypertension	160-200	100-120
vere Hypertension	Above 200	160-200

BLOOD PRESSURE LOG

NAME. ____

Date	AM		PM		Notes
	Blood pressure	Pulse	Blood pressure	Pulse	

Level of Severity	Systolic	Diastolic
Normal	120	80
Mild Hypertension	140-160	90-100
Moderate Hypertension	160-200	100-120
Severe Hypertension	Above 200	160-200

Blood Pressure Log

Name. ___________________________

Date	AM		PM		Notes
	Blood pressure	Pulse	Blood pressure	Pulse	

vel of Severity	Systolic	Diastolic
rmal	120	80
ld Hypertension	140-160	90-100
oderate Hypertension	160-200	100-120
vere Hypertension	Above 200	160-200

BLOOD PRESSURE LOG

NAME. ____

| Date | AM | | PM | | Notes |
	Blood pressure	Pulse	Blood pressure	Pulse	

Level of Severity	Systolic	Diastolic
Normal	120	80
Mild Hypertension	140-160	90-100
Moderate Hypertension	160-200	100-120
Severe Hypertension	Above 200	160-200

Blood Pressure Log

NAME. _______________________________

Date	AM		PM		Notes
	Blood pressure	Pulse	Blood pressure	Pulse	

Level of Severity	Systolic	Diastolic
Normal	120	80
Mild Hypertension	140-160	90-100
Moderate Hypertension	160-200	100-120
Severe Hypertension	Above 200	160-200

BLOOD PRESSURE LOG

NAME. ____

Date	AM		PM		Notes
	Blood pressure	Pulse	Blood pressure	Pulse	

Level of Severity	Systolic	Diastolic
Normal	120	80
Mild Hypertension	140-160	90-100
Moderate Hypertension	160-200	100-120
Severe Hypertension	Above 200	160-200

BLOOD PRESSURE LOG

NAME. _______________________

Date	AM		PM		Notes
	Blood pressure	Pulse	Blood pressure	Pulse	

el of Severity	Systolic	Diastolic
mal	120	80
d Hypertension	140-160	90-100
derate Hypertension	160-200	100-120
vere Hypertension	Above 200	160-200

BLOOD PRESSURE LOG

NAME. ____

Date	AM		PM		Notes
	Blood pressure	Pulse	Blood pressure	Pulse	

Level of Severity	Systolic	Diastolic
Normal	120	80
Mild Hypertension	140-160	90-100
Moderate Hypertension	160-200	100-120
Severe Hypertension	Above 200	160-200

BLOOD PRESSURE LOG

NAME. ____

| Date | AM | | PM | | Notes |
	Blood pressure	Pulse	Blood pressure	Pulse	

vel of Severity	Systolic	Diastolic
rmal	120	80
ld Hypertension	140-160	90-100
oderate Hypertension	160-200	100-120
vere Hypertension	Above 200	160-200

BLOOD PRESSURE LOG

NAME. ____

Date	AM		PM		Notes
	Blood pressure	Pulse	Blood pressure	Pulse	

Level of Severity	Systolic	Diastolic
Normal	120	80
Mild Hypertension	140-160	90-100
Moderate Hypertension	160-200	100-120
Severe Hypertension	Above 200	160-200

BLOOD PRESSURE LOG

NAME. ____

Date	AM		PM		Notes
	Blood pressure	Pulse	Blood pressure	Pulse	

Level of Severity	Systolic	Diastolic
Normal	120	80
Mild Hypertension	140-160	90-100
Moderate Hypertension	160-200	100-120
Severe Hypertension	Above 200	160-200

____
____
____
____
____
____
____

BLOOD PRESSURE LOG

NAME. ____

Date	AM		PM		Notes
	Blood pressure	Pulse	Blood pressure	Pulse	

Level of Severity	Systolic	Diastolic
Normal	120	80
Mild Hypertension	140-160	90-100
Moderate Hypertension	160-200	100-120
Severe Hypertension	Above 200	160-200

BLOOD PRESSURE LOG

NAME. _______________________________

Date	AM		PM		Notes
	Blood pressure	Pulse	Blood pressure	Pulse	

el of Severity	Systolic	Diastolic
mal	120	80
d Hypertension	140-160	90-100
derate Hypertension	160-200	100-120
vere Hypertension	Above 200	160-200

Blood Pressure Log

Name. ____

Date	AM		PM		Notes
	Blood pressure	Pulse	Blood pressure	Pulse	

Level of Severity	Systolic	Diastolic
Normal	120	80
Mild Hypertension	140-160	90-100
Moderate Hypertension	160-200	100-120
Severe Hypertension	Above 200	160-200

BLOOD PRESSURE LOG

NAME. ____

Date	AM		PM		Notes
	Blood pressure	Pulse	Blood pressure	Pulse	

Level of Severity	Systolic	Diastolic
Normal	120	80
Mild Hypertension	140-160	90-100
Moderate Hypertension	160-200	100-120
Severe Hypertension	Above 200	160-200

BLOOD PRESSURE LOG

NAME. ____

Date	AM		PM		Notes
	Blood pressure	Pulse	Blood pressure	Pulse	

Level of Severity	Systolic	Diastolic
Normal	120	80
Mild Hypertension	140-160	90-100
Moderate Hypertension	160-200	100-120
Severe Hypertension	Above 200	160-200

Blood Pressure Log

NAME. ____

Date	AM		PM		Notes
	Blood pressure	Pulse	Blood pressure	Pulse	

Level of Severity	Systolic	Diastolic
Normal	120	80
Mild Hypertension	140-160	90-100
Moderate Hypertension	160-200	100-120
Severe Hypertension	Above 200	160-200

BLOOD PRESSURE LOG

NAME. ____

Date	AM		PM		Notes
	Blood pressure	Pulse	Blood pressure	Pulse	

Level of Severity	Systolic	Diastolic
Normal	120	80
Mild Hypertension	140-160	90-100
Moderate Hypertension	160-200	100-120
Severe Hypertension	Above 200	160-200

BLOOD PRESSURE LOG

NAME. _______________________________________

| Date | AM | | PM | | Notes |
	Blood pressure	Pulse	Blood pressure	Pulse	

el of Severity	Systolic	Diastolic
mal	120	80
d Hypertension	140-160	90-100
derate Hypertension	160-200	100-120
ere Hypertension	Above 200	160-200

Blood Pressure Log

NAME. ____

Date	AM		PM		Notes
	Blood pressure	Pulse	Blood pressure	Pulse	

Level of Severity	Systolic	Diastolic
Normal	120	80
Mild Hypertension	140-160	90-100
Moderate Hypertension	160-200	100-120
Severe Hypertension	Above 200	160-200

BLOOD PRESSURE LOG

NAME. ____

Date	AM		PM		Notes
	Blood pressure	Pulse	Blood pressure	Pulse	

Level of Severity	Systolic	Diastolic
Normal	120	80
Mild Hypertension	140-160	90-100
Moderate Hypertension	160-200	100-120
Severe Hypertension	Above 200	160-200

BLOOD PRESSURE LOG

NAME. ____

Date	AM		PM		Notes
	Blood pressure	Pulse	Blood pressure	Pulse	

Level of Severity	Systolic	Diastolic
Normal	120	80
Mild Hypertension	140-160	90-100
Moderate Hypertension	160-200	100-120
Severe Hypertension	Above 200	160-200

Blood Pressure Log

NAME. ____

Date	AM		PM		Notes
	Blood pressure	Pulse	Blood pressure	Pulse	

Level of Severity	Systolic	Diastolic
Normal	120	80
Mild Hypertension	140-160	90-100
Moderate Hypertension	160-200	100-120
Severe Hypertension	Above 200	160-200

BLOOD PRESSURE LOG

NAME. ____

Date	AM		PM		Notes
	Blood pressure	Pulse	Blood pressure	Pulse	

Level of Severity	Systolic	Diastolic
Normal	120	80
Mild Hypertension	140-160	90-100
Moderate Hypertension	160-200	100-120
Severe Hypertension	Above 200	160-200

www.ingramcontent.com/pod-product-compliance
Lightning Source LLC
Chambersburg PA
CBHW070859250726

48662CB00003B/1457